W9-CZI-034

JUNE **1994**   JULY   AUGUST   SEPTEMBER

OCTOBER | NOVEMBER | DECEMBER | JANUARY

Path Through the Fire

WENDY ALLEN WHEELER

PATH THROUGH THE

A Cancer Story

FIRE

My thanks to my extended family and to everyone who helped me with this book. Special thanks to Jessie Schell, Stephanie Perrin, Alexandra Merrill, and Heidi Downey for their editorial help; to Angie Hurlbut and Stephanie Church for their creative design; to Betty Foster for studio space; and to Gustav Freedman for his photo.

Wheeler, Wendy
    Path Through the Fire: A Cancer Story
    ISBN 0–9666778–0–3

Design: AH Design, Angie Hurlbut and Stephanie Church

FOR MY HUSBAND, MY CHILDREN, AND THEIR PARTNERS.

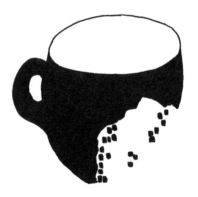

Last night (November 3, 1996, two years, four months after surgery) I woke with an image of a broken porcelain teacup, beautiful, pure white on the inside and glazed black on the outside. I was trying to put the cup back together, tiny black square by tiny black square, each piece a part of a mosaic, and, as in a jigsaw puzzle, one as important as the other and each crucial to the whole. I see this as an image for what I'm trying to do in this book, fit all the pieces together, negative and positive, that helped me keep myself together during my chemotherapy and put myself back together since then—long, intricate work. It's the first graphic image that I've had since I finished treatment two years ago. I have learned to trust my night thinking, my dreams and images. When I remember them clearly enough to draw them or write them down, I trust that they have something to tell me. I don't always know the meaning right away, but I know that the meaning will come.

Path Through the Fire

INTRODUCTION

If stories come to you, care for them. And learn to give them
away where they are needed. Sometimes a person needs a story
more than food to stay alive.

Barry Lopez, Crow and Weasel, 1990

Everyone who has had cancer has a story to tell. When I was diagnosed with breast cancer, I read everything I could find, looking for answers, looking for others who felt the same way that I did. I was particularly comforted by others' stories of their experiences.

My story came to me in images, through dreams, and through the words in my journal. I tell it here to serve my further healing and the healing of my family. If my pictures and words also help others ease their way through cancer or any other life-threatening or debilitating disease, I will be pleased.

I want to tell about the bittersweetness of the whole experience: the sickness and the hope, the terror and the unending love and support of my family and friends; the edge between rational and imaginal knowing, and, for me, the need for both.

My drawings and journal writings were critical. They mirrored and guided me through the heat, the intensity, the destructive and healing powers of chemotherapy and radiation, and led me on my particular path through the fire.

In March 1994, while taking a shower, I discovered a lump in my breast; not exactly a lump, but a tiny nodule that hadn't been there before. I immediately broke out in a cold sweat. Something was very wrong. I knew it. I frantically searched to see whether there were any other lumps, but didn't find any. I didn't have a lump like it in the other breast. By the time I got out of the shower I was in a panic. I didn't know what to do. After a while I decided that it mustn't be true. It couldn't be true. I had had a negative mammogram in September. It must be an anomaly, probably some kind of cyst that would disappear if I stopped drinking coffee. I constantly felt for the lump, believing or hoping that it would have disappeared. It didn't go away, so I went to my internist in mid-April. Thinking it was a cyst, she suggested we wait a month or two to see whether it changed. In May she ordered another mammogram. The result: "something suspicious." I was referred to an excellent general surgeon who didn't think that what she was feeling matched what she saw on the mammogram. Could I really have a tumor? Could I have cancer?

On June 3 the surgeon performed what she believed would be a routine biopsy. She had explained all the possibilities to my husband Wheel, and me, but she wasn't too concerned, so neither was I. Four hours later I came out of surgery having had a lumpectomy.

The surgeon brought Wheel into the recovery room and told us in the most straightforward but gentle way that she had removed a cyst and a small tumor underneath it. The cyst was benign. The tumor was malignant. I had cancer. I can't even describe our shock, our disbelief. Cancer happens to other people. There was no history of breast cancer in my family. I was a healthy, postmenopausal fifty-eight-year-old mother of four and grandmother of two. It couldn't be true. I was numb. I was terrified. I was incredulous. Was there a mistake? There was no mistake. I had cancer. If anyone had to give us this horrendous news, I'm grateful that it was this particular doctor. Not only is she a skilled surgeon, but she is one of the warmest, most compassionate, and loving human beings I have ever met.

3

Unfortunately, the pathology reports came back with grim news: some cancer cells were left. My "margins were not clear." I needed additional surgery to remove the remaining cancer cells and to do a lymph dissection to see if any lymph nodes were involved. June 13 was to be the day. I felt as if I were floating in unreality. Amy and Beth, our twin daughters, came home to be with Wheel and me. It was they who insisted that I ask the doctor and nurses to say only positive things during surgery and that I be allowed to listen to my CD player. Having grown up in a generation that rarely considered either the option or the benefit of patient involvement, neither of these requests would ever have occurred to me. But both requests were granted, the anaesthetist pushing the restart button on the CD player! This was the first of many lessons I was to learn during the next six months about being an advocate for my own care and treatment. Shortly after I came out of surgery and until I went home, Beth, who is a massage therapist, climbed into the bed behind me and massaged my shoulder and arm. When I left the hospital I could raise my arm above my head with very little pain. This was an auspicious beginning to my recovery and a barometer of my children's willingness to involve themselves. My family encouraged me throughout to stand up for what I knew to be important and not to assume that the doctors had all the answers.

Wheel and I had interviewed two oncologists and had chosen a woman whose upbeat office and staff appealed to us, though she herself seemed impersonal and even a bit cold. Her plan was to start with radiation and follow with chemotherapy. The pathology reports from the second surgery had not come in by the time Wheel and I went to meet the radiation oncologist. He asked us to wait in the examining room while he checked on the reports. When he returned, we could tell by his face that the news was bad. We had just met this man and he had to be the one to tell us that I had "extensive lymph involvement" and that I would have to start immediately with aggressive chemotherapy followed by radiation, the reverse of the original plan. The news was devastating. What did this mean? How could it be true? The tumor hadn't been that large, only 1.5 centimeters. I'd been feeling fine—just a little tired—and my body had been trouble-free for years. What had happened? How could this thing be eating my body without my even knowing or feeling it? So many questions. Was there a mistake? What had I done wrong? So much for living a healthy and active life. Was I going to die? The only positive note in the midst of this terrible news was this remarkable man's attitude and approach. As he gave us the report, his eyes filled with tears as did ours, and he apologized for having to tell us. He then had the grace to leave us alone while we tried to digest this news.

This was another experience with a doctor whose compassion and loving nature direct his work. The oncology nurse who administered my chemotherapy every three weeks for six months was also a real pro. I had total confidence in her. She was friendly, funny, and gentle, making the four-plus hours while the chemicals dripped into my veins not only tolerable but even occasionally amusing.

Throughout my treatment and since, my internist, my surgeon, and my radiation oncologist have been essential members of my support system and crucial to my attitude toward my cancer, always ready to answer any question, caring about me as a whole person with a life separate from disease. They are as natural and easy healers as I've met. They encouraged a positive outlook and attitude by living that way themselves. These doctors gave me facts; they didn't minimize the risks, but they didn't dwell on statistics and survival rates, and they didn't have a pessimistic perspective, though, given their practice, they certainly could have. Many in their fields do. They relieved our anxiety by explaining everything to us. There were no secrets.

My experience with doctors, however, was not always as positive. I had chosen my primary oncologist because she was a woman, and because her office was so different from some of the stark, cold, clinical offices I'd visited. She prescribed a very aggressive protocol, and I respected her as a tough and thorough clinician. She was willing to consult with other doctors about my case. She turned out, however, to be short on interpersonal skills. She seemed more attentive to me as a clinical case than as a person trying to deal with questions and fears about the disease. When we were in her office she rarely acknowledged Wheel's presence and seemed uninterested in his questions. She asked me what seemed like perfunctory personal questions and wasn't interested in hearing about any of the alternative practices that I was considering, such as vitamin supplements, acupuncture, and a low-fat diet. I often felt that I was no more than another diseased breast that needed treatment. I realized that her job was to treat me clinically, and I stayed with her because I knew I needed a competent clinician who would treat my disease aggressively. I'm grateful that she gave me the treatment she did, but I would have liked more compassion and human contact from her as my primary caregiver.

There were many decisions to make besides choosing an oncologist. Should I explore stem cell replacement, mastectomy, radiation? If I have radiation, will it, in the long run, give me more cancer? Will the lumpectomy be enough? I read many books, looking everywhere for the right answers. But I didn't even know what the questions were. I felt overwhelmed. Wheel was invaluable during doctor's appointments, reminding me of my questions and taking notes when I was too scared to hear all the details. We also talked over many of our quandaries with our children and their partners. I knew that I was not alone.

I felt as if I was on a mental and emotional roller coaster, listening to and reading information offering differing points of view, weighing alternatives, making decisions about doctors and treatment protocols while still trying to deal somehow with the shock of the two surgeries and the diagnosis. In June I began to keep a journal.

JUNE **30**

I'm exhausted—from this last month's ups and downs, from the amount of information I've had to process, the unbelievability of this cancer in my body, the doctor's appointments, the tests, the vein-pokes, the surgeries, the emotions, mine and others', the decisions—finally, yesterday, the decision about an oncologist. EXHAUSTED. Also relieved that, finally, I'll be on a course of treatment. Something will be being done. BUT, is it the right course? She talks about stem cell harvesting and bone marrow transplants. Have I chosen right? How the hell do I know? All I can go on is feelings once I've asked all the questions I know.

Today I start chemotherapy and I'm feeling as if two things are happening. 1) I'm sealing my fate and about to poison my body with harsh chemicals, changing my body composition from how it's always been to how it will always be, and 2) if I think positively, which I must, I will envision the chemo as finally something beneficent that will, drip by drip, help to counteract the poisonous cancer which has already changed and is still trying to change my body. I must think of the chemicals as healing, as

helpers—but I must think of them as more aggressive than that.
I must envision them as attacking and killing. The steady drip of
the chemo, like a heartbeat; regular, deliberate, counteracting
the wild abandon of the rapidly dividing cancer cells. I must get
inside my body and watch it do its work, be a witness to the
destruction of the stalking killer.

I hoped that the lumpectomy, chemo, and radiation would arrest the spread of the cancer, but I also wondered about the underlying cause of the cancer and what I might do to help. I felt that the doctors would attack the problem from the outside but decided that I'd better work on myself from the inside. I needed to find some areas where I could make some choices and feel some control. I refused to allow my own feelings of impotence make me fall victim to the disease. Believing that the environment probably has a lot to do with the increase in all cancers, I decided that I must do what I could to improve my personal environment, including watching my diet, exercising, resting enough, and managing stress better. I knew that I wanted to explore alternative therapies to use in conjunction with the chemo. Many people gave me advice and books to read, all of which were helpful, but there was too much to digest, and I didn't know how to decide. Should I pursue ayurvedic medicine, vitamin and mineral therapy, or a macrobiotic diet? Should I take shark cartilage? What to do about nausea and mouth sores? My oncologist seemed uninterested in any of my attempts to heal myself other than the chemo, so I didn't feel that I could count on her. I needed to find someone to help me make some decisions and coordinate my treatments.

I decided to go to a naturopathic physician for acupuncture and to have her advise me about my vitamin intake and herbal aids for liver function and immune system boosters. With so much to choose from, I finally had to trust my instincts and do what felt right to me. Throughout, I had friends who worked on me to release blocked energy. I subscribed to alternative therapy journals. I had massage and connective tissue work. A group of women from Maine sent me a "healing quilt" that they had made, each woman creating a square that represented healing to her. Wheel wrapped me in it for each chemo treatment, and often I slept under it. I had a friend who, whenever I had a question about anything, would post the question on the Internet and send me the responses. Having tried one breast cancer support group I decided not to join one, because I didn't want to hear everyone else's horror stories about recurrences and treatments that didn't work. Instead, I chose to be with my family and friends, who, though confused and sad, had positive attitudes. I also met some other women with breast cancer who had basically upbeat attitudes despite often feeling scared or angry. It was a relief to be able to talk about being afraid that we might die or that the chemotherapy might kill us before the cancer did. We did cry, we did feel angry. We helped each other keep going, and we laughed.

Laughter was and is essential to my healing. I met one friend when I went to a "Look Good, Feel Better" makeup and makeover session sponsored by the American Cancer Society. Chemo had caused me to lose all of my hair. I had bought a wig that I never wore because I hated it. Instead, I wore scarves and turbans and felt comfortable in them. There were five or six of us there and I offered to be the model for the makeup and wig part. I took off my turban and sat there, bald as a baby. The others had their proper wigs on. Gradually the other women removed their wigs and we relaxed. We laughed pretty hard at some of the wigs the "hair lady" put on me, and when I left that meeting, I felt as if I was wearing at least an inch of makeup. I could hardly open my eyes! My new friends and I would get together for lunch and share stories that no one else could possibly appreciate about some of the grosser side effects of chemo and radiation. I still laugh about one lunch when we were regaling each other with stories. We were laughing uproariously when my friend got too hot and, without thinking, whipped off her wig. The looks on people's faces, including that of our waitress, were priceless! I also remember the time I invited some of our friends for a birthday party and a couple of the women and I decided to dress up. We ended up wearing my turbans, wild earrings, and makeup and came downstairs singing and dancing and calling ourselves "The Chemo Chics!" All of these experiences helped to lighten the load and to act as antidotes to the grimmer side of the treatment, giving me a feeling of some balance and helping me not become a victim of the disease.

9

DRAWINGS AND JOURNAL WRITING

I had read about the use of art therapy during chemotherapy and I had known for a long time about the value of visualization, but I discovered for myself the value of art and image making in my own healing. Two days after my first treatment I had been very nauseated. Just before I fell asleep, I had an image of myself wearing a miner's hat. I was walking through my body and the light was guiding the chemicals to the cancer cells. The nausea subsided. The next night the image was of white rats wandering through my insides eating the cancer cells. Behind them little white mice picked up what the rats missed. The nausea subsided briefly. Several times, when I was feeling nauseated, I would get an image of yellow or pale peach light that would envelop me, and the nausea would diminish. While it didn't always work, I was learning for myself about the power of visualization and imagemaking.

Interestingly, the minute I started chemotherapy I seemed to let go of much of my thinking function and move into the other side of my brain, to the imaginal realm. It's as if once I knew a decision had been made and something tangible was being done, I let go of having any notion of controlling anything external. I flew for refuge into my imagination, letting my unconscious and sentient self lead me. I put my rational self in the hands of the chemicals, the doctors, and the fates. I didn't know how to do much more on the conscious level. What I did do was keep a daily journal about my experience. The combination of imagemaking and journal writing was comforting, often energizing, and a powerful way for me to express my feelings. However, it was a bittersweet experience; there was such a contrast between the chemo, the fear that my immune system might give way entirely and never recover, and the often blissful feeling of floating in my senses that I had when I did the drawings. The sickness I was feeling seemed to force my body and mind to slow down enough to allow the rest of me to wake up.

I've been spending the past 15 years learning about the creative parts of myself—literally through painting, pottery, and writing. Now I need to delve deeper into the part of my soul that knows how to begin the creation. I need to talk to that part of me and engage that part of me in this healing. I think the healing part of me has to do with color and light, and I need to somehow summon those aids in this mission.

Where's my sense of outrage? Where, even, is my anger? I need to ENGAGE. I feel as if I'm numb still, going along with the diagnosis, doing what I'm supposed to be doing, being a "good" patient, learning a bit as I go along—ready to deal, ready to accept hair loss, fatigue, nausea—half-heartedly looking into alternatives. I hear others' outrage. I think I'm managing with a veil or semi-permeable shield around me so that I don't feel, protecting myself from my own feelings as well as others'. I need to move on from this accepting place, this numbing, somewhat martyred place, this non-feeling victim place into a place of action—action even in the quiet.

Maybe I need to cure this cancer with my own creative fire—to burn out the poison, the cancer, the tumor. Maybe the image, the visualization for me is about fire, which includes rage, outrage, passion, and sensuality, destruction as well as cleansing, healing and transformation; an image of creation and destruction and finding a way to live in that balance. I know the danger of falling into the destructive, lethargic, sorry-for-myself part of me and dying there. I know this battle is not only between the actual cancer and the chemicals but between the intrapsychic killing cancer and the creative healer in me. I will take early morning time and some other time during the day for quiet, for meditation, for listening to music and drawing or painting. I'll get myself new art supplies—good ones—and through music and color I'll take myself into my own feeling.

I had no idea what my images would look like, but I knew that I wanted them to be contained in circles—mandalas. I didn't know much about mandalas, but when I looked up the definition, I found that, among other things, they are "graphic mystical symbols of the universe." The decision to put all my images inside circles was a decision made instinctively. It was something I just knew.

For the first time in my life I went into an art store and knew exactly what I wanted. Usually I'm so overwhelmed with choices that I can manage only to buy a pencil or pen. This time, having decided that I needed to get new art supplies, I came out in fifteen minutes with magic markers, crayons, colored pencils, a paintbrush, and a giant blank book.

During the next six months I made thirty-seven drawings, twenty-seven of which are reproduced here. I made them because I had to make them. The drawing was an imperative from deep inside me. I would sit down, spread all my colors out in front of me, open my book, and make a circle. Sometimes I'd have a dream or an image in the night and I would turn it into a drawing, or a vivid image would come to me during the day. Other times I would sit down, make the circle, look at all my colors and wait for a color to say "start with me." Then I would let the colors do the work. Each time I would feel a surge of adrenaline, of health, of warmth and excitement. Oblivious of anything going on around me, I would often spend two to three hours doing a drawing and not be aware of time passing. The slowness centered me, pulled me back from the frenzy in my head and the frenzy of the work I envisioned the chemo was doing. Sometimes music played in my head and I would hum the whole time. Sometimes there were words about the image, and for some the meaning came after the drawing. I felt as if I were connected to myself deep inside and out somewhere in the universe. No matter how sick I felt, how angry or sad I was, the drawing was soothing and true. I was expressing exactly where I was. Most of the drawings came from so deep inside me that, looking at them, I can still feel the feelings I had while drawing them. Sometimes I'd feel sad, sometimes elated, sometimes angry, sometimes overwhelmed. The drawing was one part of the creative process going on inside me. Equally important was my journal. Together they tell the whole story.

I can't write about those six months of treatment without describing a crucial event that involves my family and their loyalty. I had started a very aggressive dosage of chemotherapy and knew that, among other side effects, my hair would fall out. I had been thinking a lot about what it would be like to have no hair and how horrible it would be to find clumps of hair on the pillow every morning, so I decided that, whenever my hair started to fall out, I would shave it all off. After I made this decision, I had a dream about Joan of Arc, girding herself for battle. I was clear about what I needed to do.

The year before, we had arranged for our four children (aged twenty-eight to thirty-three) and their partners to be with us in July at our beach house to celebrate my husband's sixtieth birthday. Four of them would be coming from as far away as Los Angeles and Washington, D.C. Also, as a surprise, our goddaughter was coming from Maine and a dear friend was coming from Australia. This was going to be a very special occasion, made even more poignant since my diagnosis. I needed them. Wheel needed them.

I think my hair may start falling out when the kids are here next week, and I want to make my head shaving a ritual, a spiritual event. I'm thinking about the act as an assertive move on my part to ready myself for battle—to do my part in this fight. I have the strongest, most powerful chemicals going into my system from the outside to fight the battle. I need to make as strong and powerful a move from the inside to balance the onslaught of the chemicals so we can attack the enemy from two fronts. So I need to pay careful attention to how I ready myself, and I want my family to participate in this readying— sort of like warrior handmaidens—men and women—to add thrust to my strength in making this move. I know that what I'm needing to do is engage as a balancer in this destructive war against destruction where killer is pitted against killer. What I need for balance so I don't annihilate myself is the strength of my own creative force fire—quiet and just as deadly as it is lifegiving.

15

On July 14, Wheel and I drove back to Connecticut for my second chemo treatment, leaving the children at the beach and intending to return that night. Unfortunately, my white count was very low. My oncologist said I would have to have daily GCSF (Neupogen) shots to bring my count up to a level where they could continue to give me the chemo and that I would have to have those shots in her office. She insisted that there was no alternative. She said she couldn't give me the medication to take back with me, and my insurance, she said, wouldn't cover the shots given in another state. That meant that I would have to stay in Connecticut indefinitely. She asked me nothing about my family and made no attempt to understand why it was so important to me to get back to the beach. I was devastated. I knew I needed the Neupogen. I also needed my children's love and support and they needed to see how I was doing. Some of them hadn't seen me since my diagnosis, and this was the only time we could all be together. I felt trapped, helpless, and very angry. This woman who was supposed to be helping me was not interested in helping me find a solution to this dilemma.

With no apparent help from the doctor, Wheel and I spent the rest of the day on the phone trying to find a way to get the medication. The children and friends at the beach tried to find a nurse or doctor who would take care of me there. They even offered to pool their resources and help us pay the $150 per shot if we could find the Neupogen. Late in the afternoon, during a phone conversation with my oncologist, she accused me of not taking my cancer seriously enough. I was tired and frustrated, and her attitude enraged me. I felt the heat rising inside me and I screamed at her for quite some time. How could she accuse me of not taking my cancer seriously enough? I was the one with the cancer—not she. I was dead serious. But I happen to believe that being with people who love you and support you is equally important medicine and what did she know about my personal needs anyway, etc. I followed up that phone call the next day with a letter further explaining my outburst.

After I told the oncology nurse that we were willing to pay for the medication, she finally found a solution. She called Connecticut Home Therapeutics, where she had once worked, and found that they would send someone to our house with a supply of Neupogen that our insurance company would cover. That person would teach me how to give myself the shots. I didn't know at the time how important being able to give myself these daily shots would be to my emotional and physical sense of independence and control. The next day we returned to the shore for the reunion and the birthday party. Such a simple solution, and one that needn't have been so traumatic had the doctor been more empathetic and willing to help.

During the birthday party, my daughter-in-law Deb gave me an extraordinary "power necklace" that she had made with objects collected from all my siblings and children. She'd asked each of them to send her an object that they believed held power or represented strength in some way. I was deeply moved by her generosity, love, and support and knew that whenever I wore it I would have the strength and spirit of all those people with me. I wore that necklace every day and during all chemo treatments and never felt alone.

My hair did start to fall out at the end of that week, and, with the encouragement of my children, I decided to carry out my plan. For the haircutting ceremony I had brought scissors and electric clippers. I brought poems to read at the beginning. Unknown to me, my son Daniel, who for years has worn his hair in a long ponytail, had decided that when I shaved my head, he would shave his. The day my hair started falling out, he disappeared and reappeared with his hair one inch long. I dressed in a beautiful caftan that I had brought for the occasion and put my power necklace on. Deb put on some music, Beth held a mirror so I could watch, and Wheel held my hand throughout. I read my poems and asked each of them to cut a section of my hair. Then Daniel said that he'd like to shape the rest with the clippers, the same ones I had used to cut his hair when he was young. He did it so lovingly that I felt as if I was being re-created. When he was finished, I looked in the mirror and saw a hairless stranger. At first I frightened myself. I didn't look like anyone I'd ever seen before. But African music from *Serafina!* was playing, and suddenly I was dancing, and then we were all dancing. I felt free. I'd taken charge of one aspect of my life, had refused to be a victim to many "bad hair days," and had shared this moving experience with my family. It was a critical time for all of us. Cancer is a family disease and one that makes everyone feel helpless. This was a moment when we didn't feel helpless and we didn't feel alone. I learned a lot about the value of a ritual that is born of the moment, not of some prescribed notion. It will remain embedded in my heart as one of the pivotal moments in my recovery and as one of the ways we found together to healthfully integrate this crisis into our lives.

This was the only time when we as a whole family were physically together during my treatment, but their presence and support was constant. Each member supported in his/her own characteristic way. Amy and Beth called often, came home for treatments, lit twenty-four-hour candles, and sent me cards and messages. Daniel and Maggie brought us T-shirts with "Team Creaky" on the back and a picture of Wheel and me on the front. (Creaky is a nickname they've had for me for years.) My daughter-in-law Maggie lit candles, built altars, and had prayers said and songs sung for me. She stayed in constant contact. My son Andrew tried unsuccessfully to teach me to use a bong to smoke the marijuana that my brother had given me for nausea, another hilarious event as I didn't seem to be able to light a lighter and inhale at the same time without burning my fingers. Andrew and Daniel called often. My sisters and brother and their spouses were in constant touch with us, being careful not to overdo or overtax us. I really felt held. In fact, I was buoyed by the constancy and support of many, many friends around the world who called me, prayed for me, sent cards and flowers, and lit candles. Although I was frightened and sick, I felt cradled by their love. I know that this support was essential to my healing.

Wheel deserves a medal. He was constant beyond measure, unendingly supportive, fiercely protective, and tenderly loving. He fended off callers in a most gentle way, helped me with each decision, helped me give myself shots, and cooked for me. He came to every chemotherapy appointment, often wearing my necklace through the parking garage, up the elevator and into the doctor's office, so that I'd be sure to have it for the treatment. He covered me in the healing quilt and sat holding my hand through the whole time. He accepted all of my varied moods, including the most irrational panics and rages. He held me in my fear and loved me throughout. I worried about him, his feelings and his dreams. I don't think I could have done it if it hadn't been for him.

The mood roller coaster of the six months of nine chemotherapy treatments is best described by the sequence of my drawings and journal writings. The original drawings were made in an 11 x 14-inch sketch book. With the exception of six of the thirty-seven drawings, all were contained within a circle made with a 9-inch dinner plate. The reproductions in this book, therefore, are considerably reduced in size. The journal entries were either the impetus for or the result of the drawings.

20

What is happening inside me is a tossup, a challenge, a war between the killing cancer and the destructive killer chemicals. I need to find a healing balance inside myself while this war goes on.

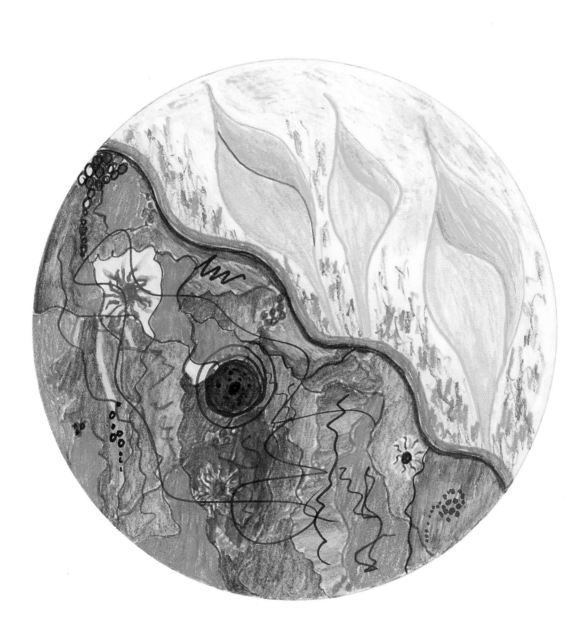

22

I'm feeling in an ESSENTIAL part of myself, uncluttered, focused and utterly simple, sort of as if I were connected to my own umbilicus, or by my own umbilicus, to a pure, unadulterated, otherworldly light space. I'm remembering the other day sitting by the pond with my friend and talking about the love, support, and sustenance I was feeling from all sides. I looked up at the blue, blue sky, put my arms out and said, "It's as if all that blue skylight, warm and enveloping, is coming out of my belly button in a straight, clear, dark filament, with intention, leading me to my next step." After all, what is the umbilicus but the thread, the connection between the infant, the soul, and the mother— the life-giving, nurturing, loving mother? So I'm feeling as if this mandala work, this reconnection with my own creative fire is connecting me to the GREAT MOTHER in me and in that outer ethereal, forever space. What is that but the experience of the core—of the essence?

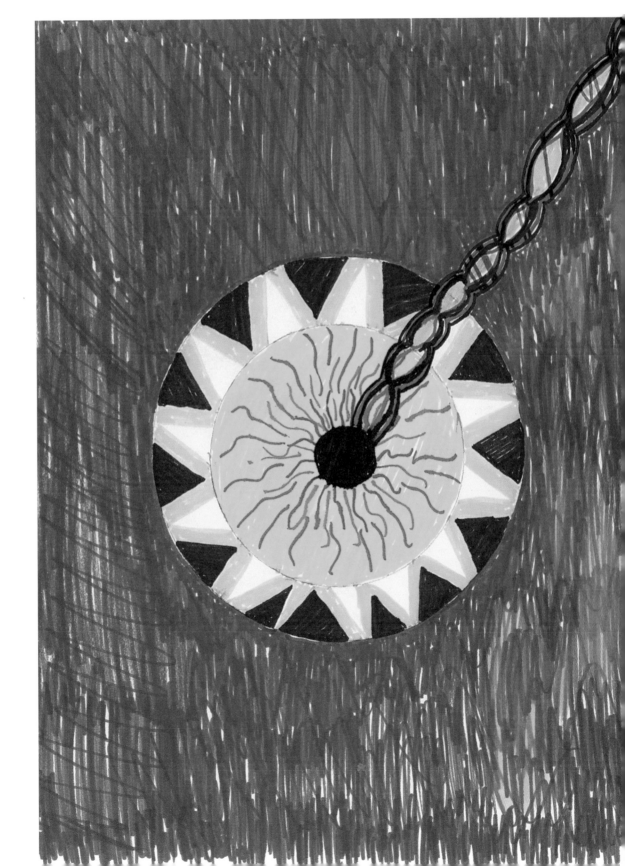

At the shore—walking and swimming and realizing, once again, that this is the beach I take myself to, in my mind's eye, whenever I want to feel quiet and peaceful. And here I am, out of fantasy and into the real thing. The water is clear, supple, and supportive and I have a lot of breath and energy for swimming. What a gift this day is!

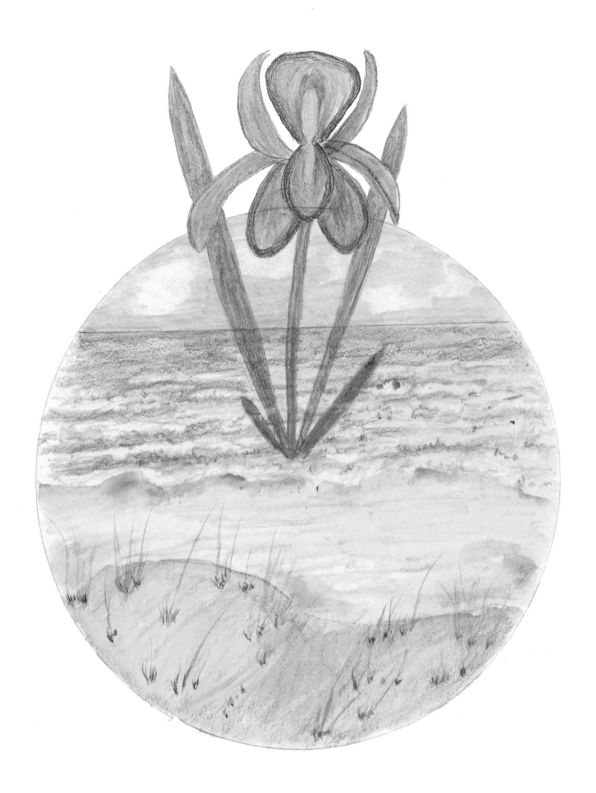

Shadow | JULY **11**

A dream in the night of two huge black wings, ominous, hovering. I knew when I woke that it was the shadow, the dark side of the peacefulness of the day before—a reminder of the seriousness of this illness. When I drew this, the wings didn't seem as dark and scary as they had. Rather, they were strong and protective, and the circle in the middle, a recurring theme, is my essence, my soul.

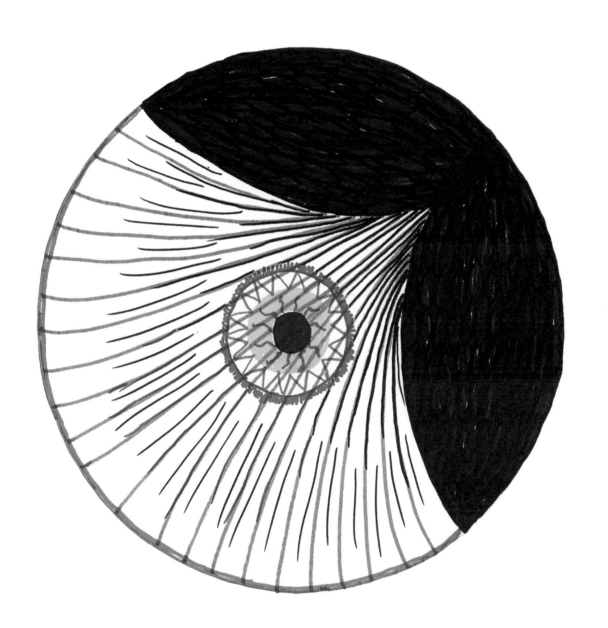

Amy's and Beth's twenty-eighth birthdays. I remember the day of their birth so well—and how grateful I am for those two caring, loving, warm, attentive, smart, and assertive women in my life. They have brought me so much joy... I can't imagine what it would be like for someone without such a loving and supportive family. I can't imagine the loneliness...

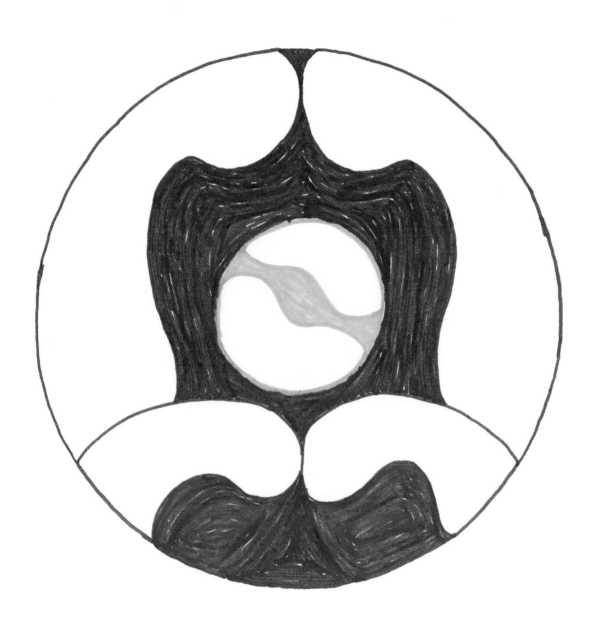

Totally furious at my oncologist who has, among other things, told me that she doesn't think I'm taking this cancer seriously enough! I have to start taking daily Neupogen shots to bring my white count up. She has threatened not to let me go back to the shore where my whole family is to celebrate my husband's birthday and doesn't seem at all interested in helping me find a way to do that. I feel as if I'm nothing to her but a diseased breast or a receptacle for her chemicals. The least she could do is treat me like a PERSON WHO HAS ANOTHER LIFE BESIDES CANCER!!!! I feel insulted and as if I've been treated like a child. She knows nothing of my family and how I need them.

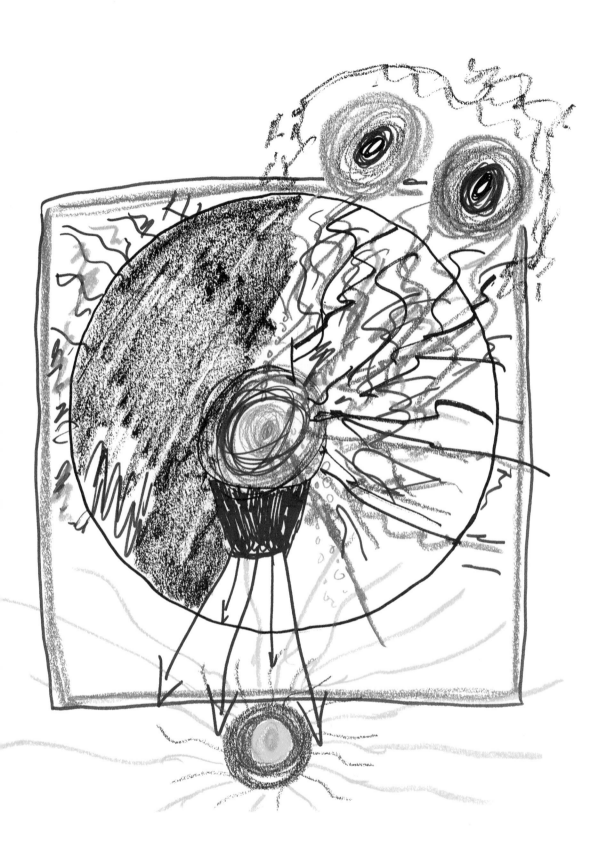

A week with all my children and their partners, our goddaughter, and a wonderful friend from Australia to celebrate my husband's sixtieth birthday. I planned it a year ago, of course having no idea how much I would need these good people myself. In the center, a feeble drawing of the incredible necklace my daughter-in-law made for me, with power/strength objects she'd collected from all my family.

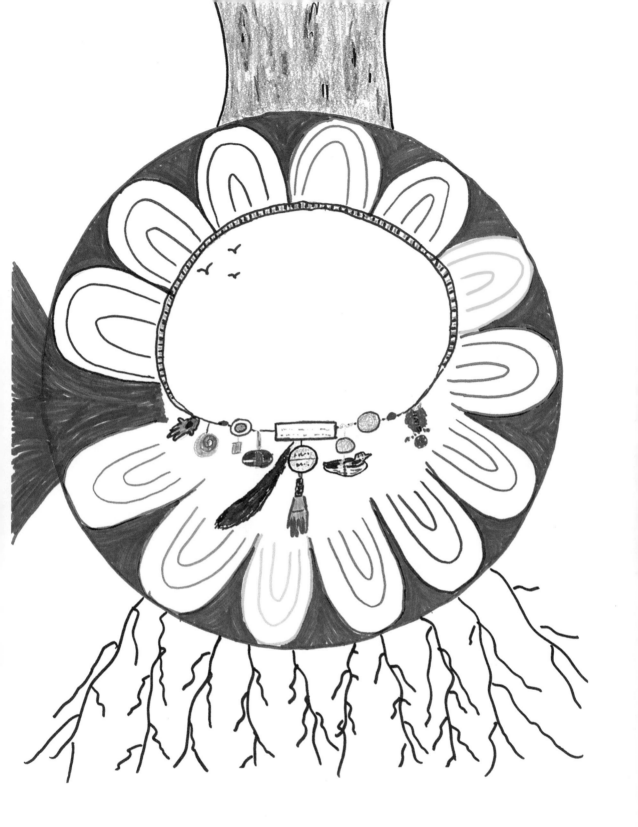

34

In and out of nausea. I've lost the illusion that I have control over anything. It doesn't really matter, on one level anyway, how you live your life, how well you take care of yourself, what a "good" person you are, etc. The design is in someone else's hands and has been all along. Feeling bombarded and feeling sad about my poor body which has served me so well and so trouble-free for so many years. I feel as if now it's full of foreign matter, foreign to it and to me. Hot flashes, depression.

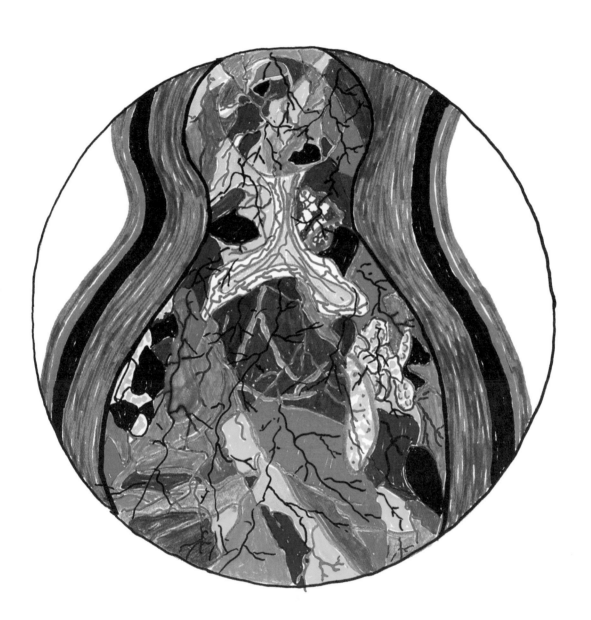

Extremely uncomfortable—the sores on my tongue are the worst, making it hard to chew, swallow, and spit. The ones on my lip make it hard to open and close my mouth. I'm sick of this! No one seems to know what to do to make them go away. I'm so goddamned tired of taking medication, vitamins, swallowing specially prepared teas, eating only foods that won't hurt my mouth, watching this, watching that. I'm beginning to feel like a sick person—not someone with a life-threatening illness but a SICK PERSON who has to be forever taking stuff, worrying about stuff, wondering if ANYONE REALLY KNOWS WHAT THE HELL IS GOING ON.

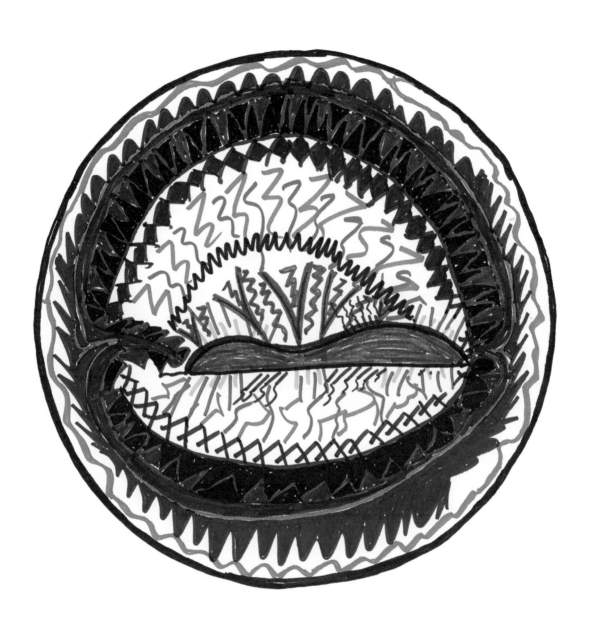

My friend Sarah came all the way from Cleveland to do some healing energy work on me. We talked a lot about visualization, healing, and power animals, and then she worked on me. I felt myself unblocking, and it felt as if my blood was rushing around my body. I could simultaneously see and feel this powerful and colorful image of the energy traveling around my body in a figure 8 pattern. The energy entered my body in the form of tiny, shiny red cells, swirled around, and, as they moved through, they became a rich, deep purple.

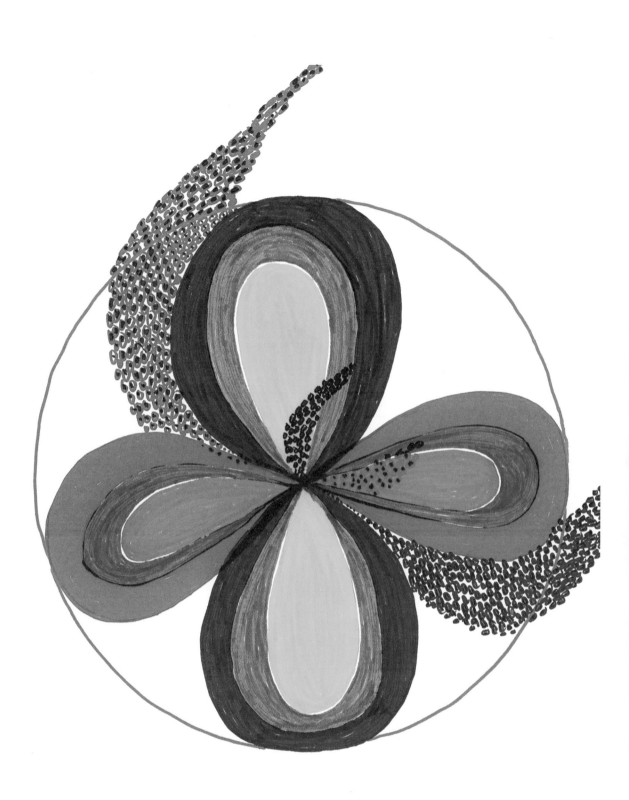

I feel confused and scared and alone—alone even though I have this incredible husband and family and friends who love me. When it comes to this fear, I really am alone and no matter what I do to heal myself, no matter how many resources I have, I'm still at the mercy of these doctors and the fates. When I go back to sleep, I have this image: a clear light-blue cylinder in which is my life force, moving constantly up and down, up and down. Lying on top of the cylinder is a giant mother cheetah who simply stares out at the world. I know that she's there to protect my life force and won't let anyone harm it. She doesn't have to do anything or fight anyone. She's just there and that's enough. She'll be aggressive if she has to, but no one's going to meddle with her.

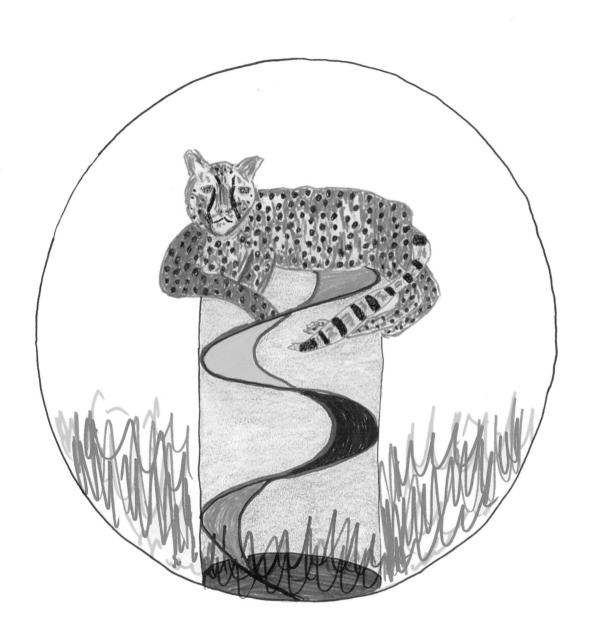

I go to bed and can't sleep. For the first time since I started chemo, I'm restless right at the start rather than in the middle of the night. I realize I'm afraid. I'm afraid I'm being experimented with, that no one really knows how much chemo to give me, that maybe I'm already fried from the chemo, that maybe the cancer's in my brain. What about the rash under my arm and the increased numbness under that left arm? Do I have an infection? How do I find out? I'm so filled with anxiety that I'm feeling crazy. I get up and write. What am I feeling? Anything? A kind of dullness, emptiness, detachment. My head and my body don't feel connected, and my body doesn't feel as if it belongs to me. I feel the nausea, the headaches, and the mouth sores, but I understand nothing. What do they mean when they talk about the survivors being the ones who have the will—no, the impera- tive—to survive? Do I have this? I'm not at all sure I do. I am a series of sensations. Will I survive? Do I care if I do? Pain and emptiness. I go back to bed and I'm cold, so I curl up in a ball, hugging myself. I waken later with my arms still around me and a warm yellow light bathing me, and I am calm.

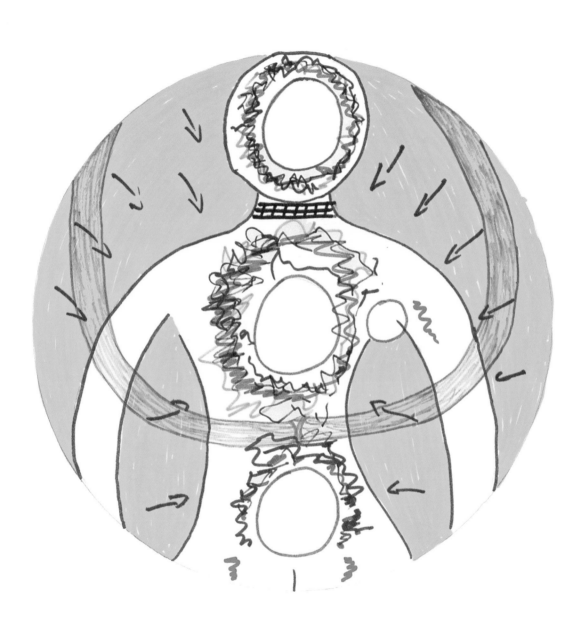

44

Fourth treatment—felt different going into this treatment—anxious all week prior to it. The nurse had trouble getting the needle into my vein. I was afraid the chemicals were going in wrong. When the nurse left, I started to cry and cried all through the session. Wheel sat with me, holding my hand and loving me. We have a picture in our bedroom of a mother cheetah protecting her little baby. The mother cheetah showed up in another drawing. I felt small and utterly vulnerable, like the baby cheetah. When I told Wheel that, he told me to let myself feel that way, he would be my mother cheetah.

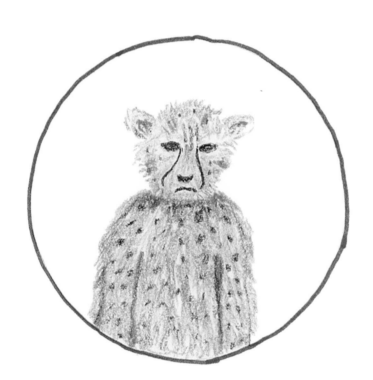

The night of the fourth treatment—an image. Before I went to sleep I asked the universe for any messages that I needed to hear, and behold—an image of St. George came to me and said, "Don't try to slay the dragon. The dragon is your heart and is where you live and your heart leads you."

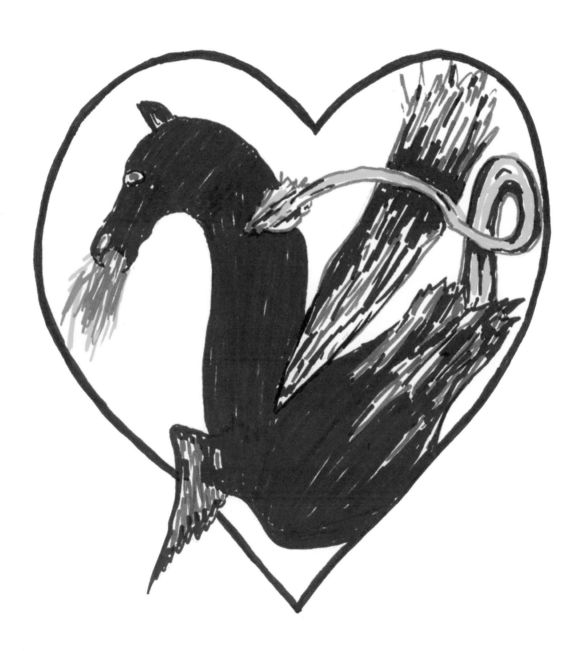

Blood test indicates low red count—anemic—not so low as to warrant a transfusion but doctor a little concerned. My friend Suzanne was doing some energy work on me, trying to free up the blockages in my energy pathways. She said that maybe the red cells were confused with so much happening to them. I immediately got an image of thousands of little red-coated soldiers walking around, bumping into each other, dazed and confused. She suggested I tell them that I understand their confusion, that there are a lot of things going on, and that I'd like them to get back to their work. They immediately (some slowly) come to attention. Later, I get the image of a lone soldier who's in the trenches of my marrow with a shovel, digging and digging in the same place. When I ask him what he's doing, he says, "Just turning it over, giving it air to breathe."

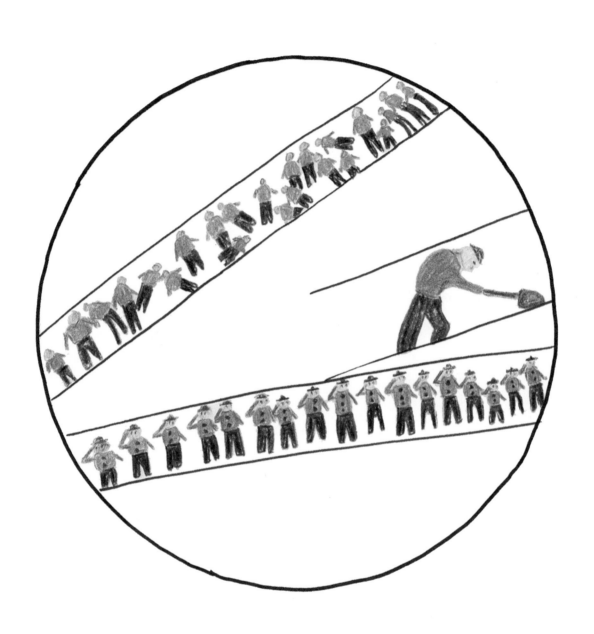

I've felt really down today—had a liver ultrasound in the morning. So much going on in my body that I can't feel and so don't understand. Without much reassurance from my oncologist, I don't know whether I'm in danger with my low red blood count and liver function. I'm also wrestling with the decision about whether to have a mastectomy at the end of chemo to avoid radiation, or if, given my extensive lymph involvement, I even have a choice. All this confuses me and makes me sad. I take a walk in the woods, and when I see a patch of sunlight way ahead, I know instinctively that I need to stand in it for a while. The sun seems to be shining there just for me, so I stand in it with my eyes closed and rest in the warmth. When I open my eyes I notice a particular tree with a split trunk and I know it's a symbol of the choices I'm trying to make: mastectomy/radiation; allopathic/naturopathic. It's about balance and going in two directions at once. I think about Yogi Berra's remark, "If you come to a fork in the road, take it." I realize that, rather than baffle myself with the choices, I need to explore both trunks of the tree in order to make a good decision.

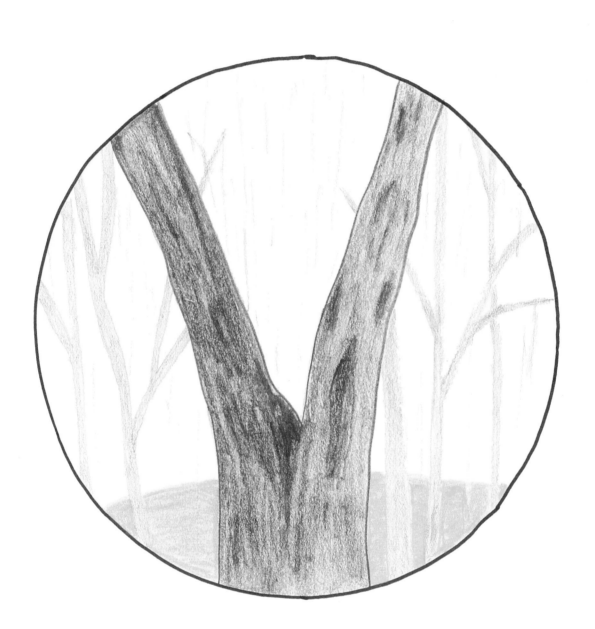

Woke this morning with an image of the "chemo cycle." I started with the pencil line drawing like a graph. At the left side, a treatment, then feeling worse and worse the next week, then feeling a little better, then much better the third week, and then starting all over again. I felt the need to trace the lines with my pencil and, as I continued, eventually, wanted some color and found, by the end, as the lines became less and less entangled and more colorful, that in fact the original line had been transformed into a kind of flower. The chemo cycle has become a cycle of transformation—the balance, again, of destruction and creation.

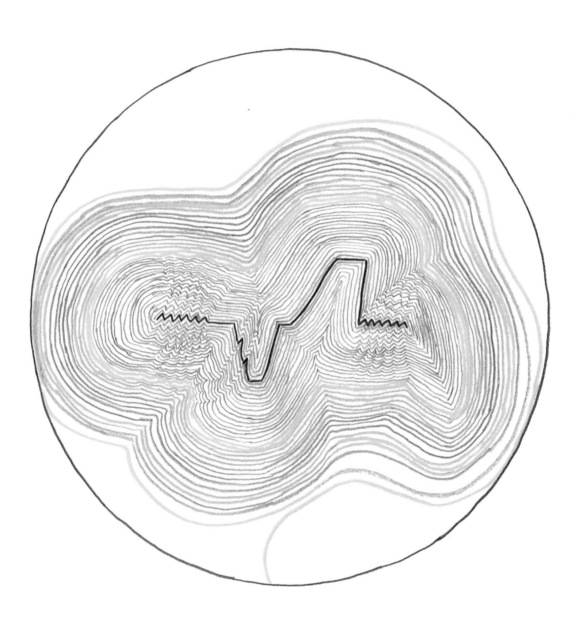

Woke with the image of me as a solitary oak tree on a hill, then of me in the form of the giant maple tree outside our house with most of its leaves on the ground but a few hanging on at the top. I have been thinking about my treatment coming up tomorrow and wondering whether my body has the strength to withstand it. My vein has hardened from the chemo. Can it take the rest of the treatments? Also, I'm realizing that there are only a few treatments left.

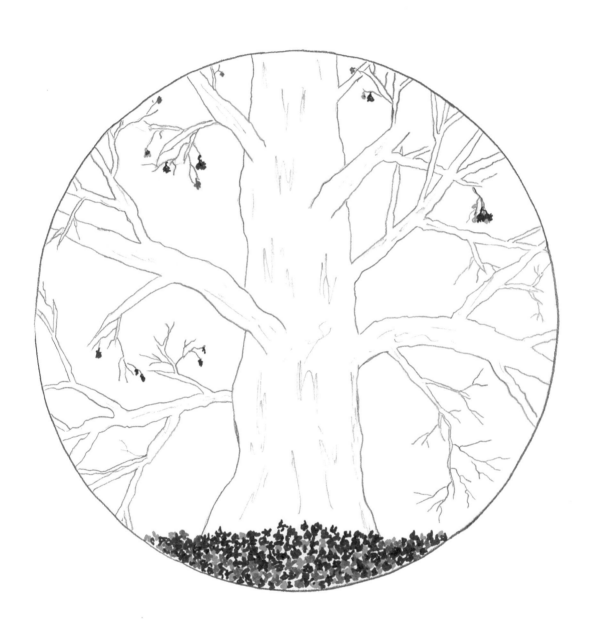

Burning sensation in my mouth and throat—headache, some nausea. Hot burning sensation all through my body. I'm on fire! What must I look like on the inside?

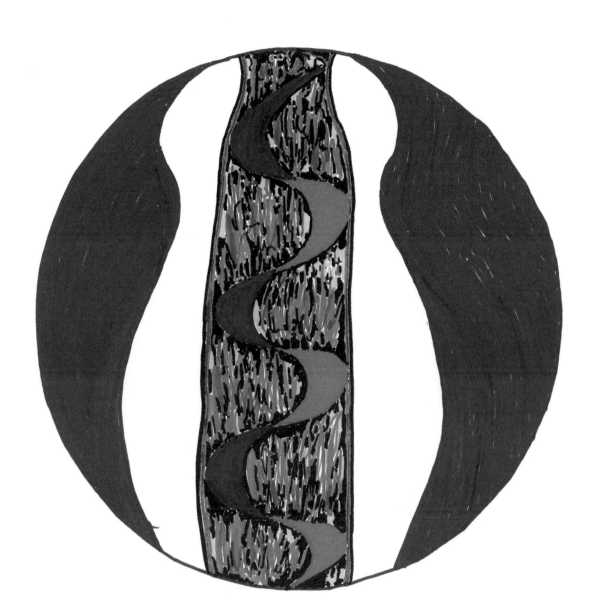

I'm thinking about the end of chemo coming up pretty soon. I've been in the very dark, both in my unknowing and in my fear. As time has gone on, the dark has lightened some as I've accepted the facts and as I've learned more about what's happening to me. The image comes to me in the night and is about moving very gradually from the dark into more light. Then I see that there are two golden wings or hands protecting me by surrounding the dark, and I'm not afraid.

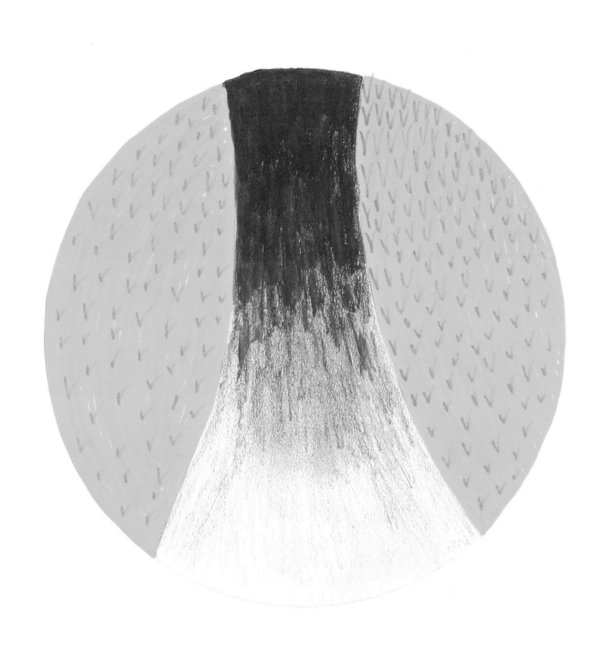

Three days later another image comes in which the golden wings or hands open up and what's left is a kind of grayness but it's open, as if the wings had opened to let me see. I feel as if I'm in the shadows but able to look out.

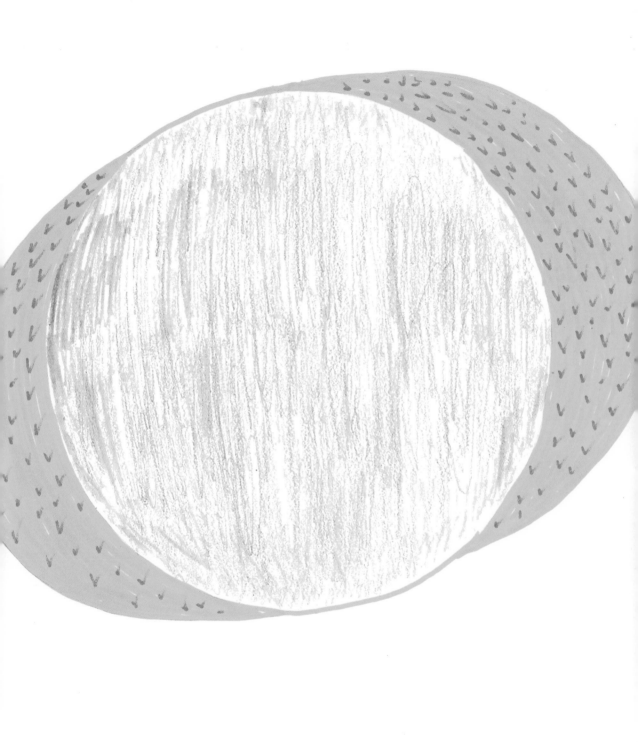

I wake up scared. I'm letting in some of the numbers, some of the statistics. When I do that, I feel very vulnerable. I know that I could end up on either side of the statistical ledger, but this morning I let the bleak side in. An image comes to me of a big black ball, totally black, totally dark. The black starts to ooze out of the bottom of the ball. It is a very scary image, in fact an image of terror. As I realize that it is an image of terror, and, as I'm feeling its impact, the next image comes in.

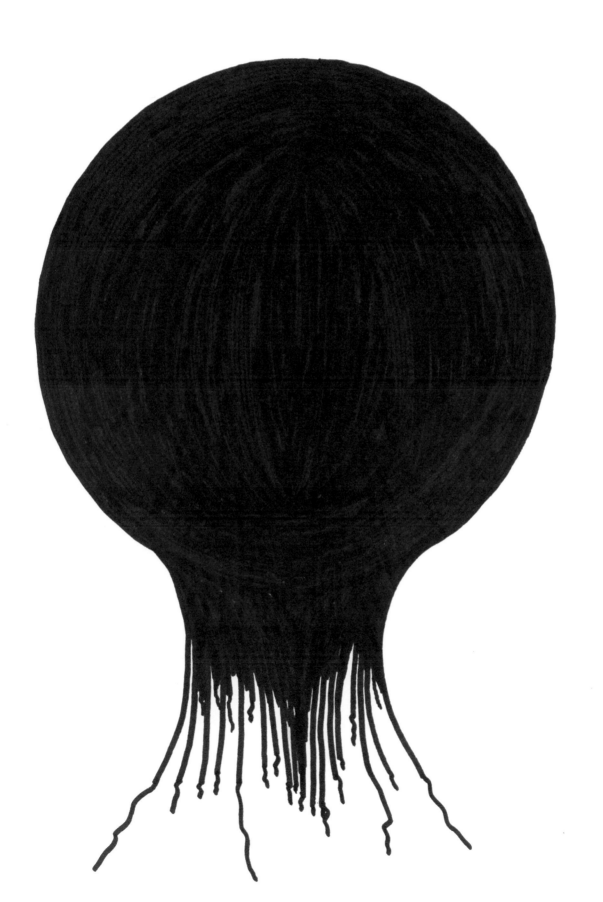

64

The black ball of terror has become transparent with a flame or a beautiful fiery filament showing through it. Golden hands (as in previous images) hold the ball, which now sits in a black dish. The phrase "cupped in the hands of" comes to me, and I suddenly feel very peaceful.

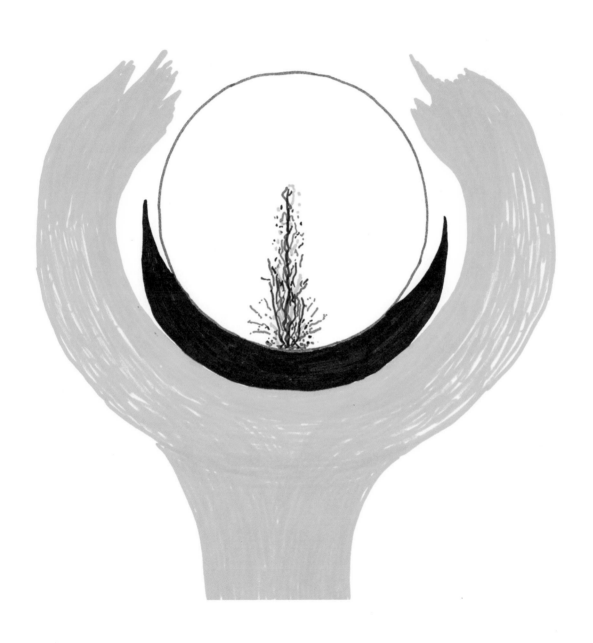

Dream after a bad day of not being able to remember much or think clearly—trouble finding words and keeping thoughts together… fear of metastasis to my brain. Is there a message here? Should I refuse the last treatment? In the dream I'm in a subway station in a foreign country. I'm looking for the subway that will take me to the station at the end of the line. I'm standing next to one of the trolleys and suddenly, by some magnetic force, I'm plastered up onto it. My whole body is lying against it. The subway starts to move toward the tunnel in front of it. I think I must get myself off the trolley or I'm going to be crushed in the tunnel. I'm in a kind of hypnotic state and feel as if I can't get myself off. I'm going to die. I make one last incredibly difficult attempt to pull my head away and it works. I pop off the trolley just before it enters the tunnel. I realize as I'm sitting on the platform that in a few seconds my head would have smashed into the wall. When I wake I know that this is about my ambivalence about the last treatment, wondering if it will kill me before the cancer can, and I wonder whether I should even go through with it.

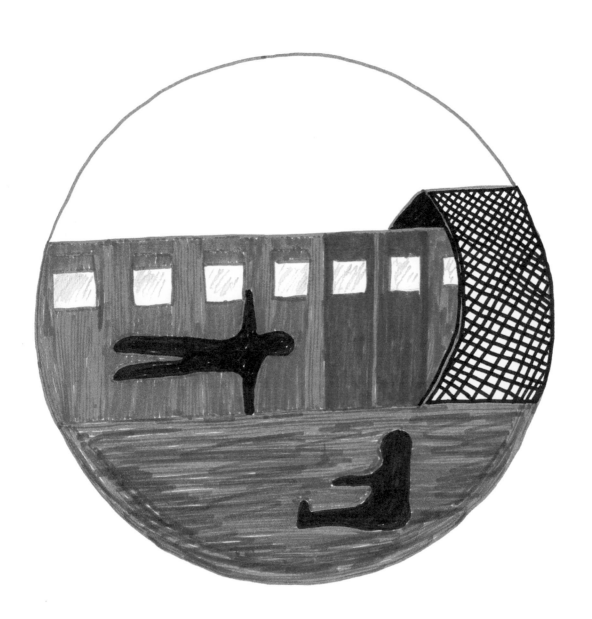

Last One—

DECEMBER **27**

The bouquet generously given me by my oncologist after my last treatment—sick as I'm feeling, here are all my favorite flowers and they're so full of life! I've made it through all the treatments and am still alive!

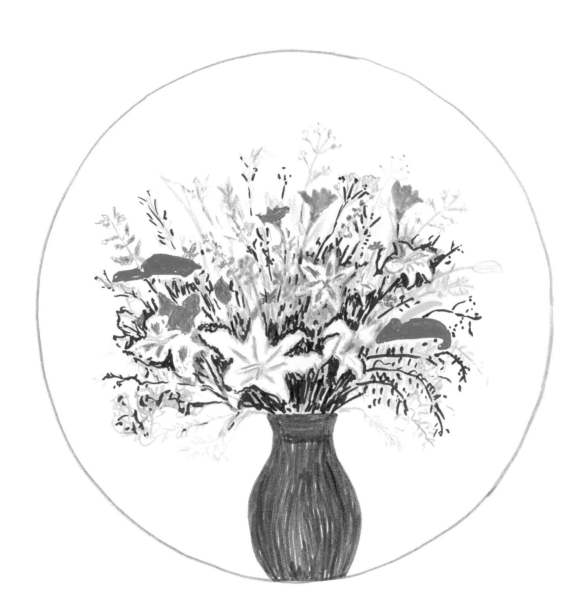

JANUARY **12**

One and a half weeks after last chemo treatment and before
radiation, I'm at Woman's Way, a women's personal growth
workshop which I've co-led for seventeen years. I'm dancing in a
circle of women, all of whom are wearing colorful long scarves
over their heads. I close my eyes and put myself in the middle of
the circle, feel the energy all around me, and imagine that all
the dancing around me is a death dance to the cancer cells.

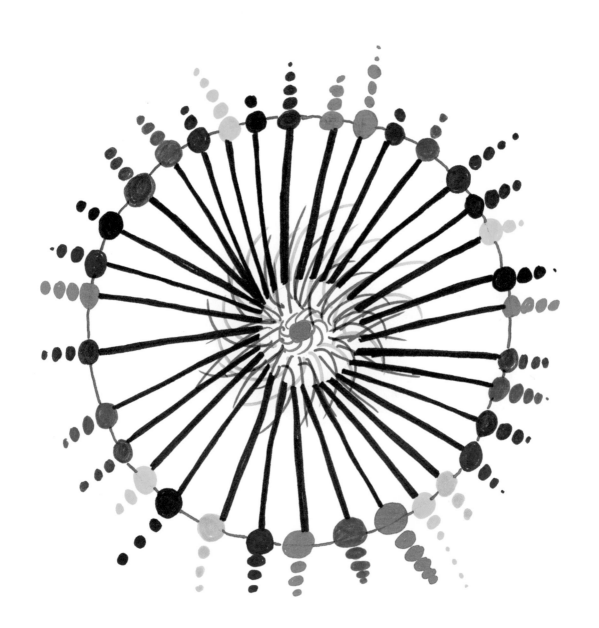

72

During the chemo I was coping, dealing with nausea and fatigue and fear. I seem to have moved to another, deeper level of comprehension and feeling. I'm feeling sadness, grief without words, a buildup and overflowing of tears which have been waiting to flow. At the workshop we have woven a beautiful web that I think of as the web of life and interconnectedness. I dream a black, shiny bird, wings outstretched under the web. It feels like the shadow of death in the midst of life.

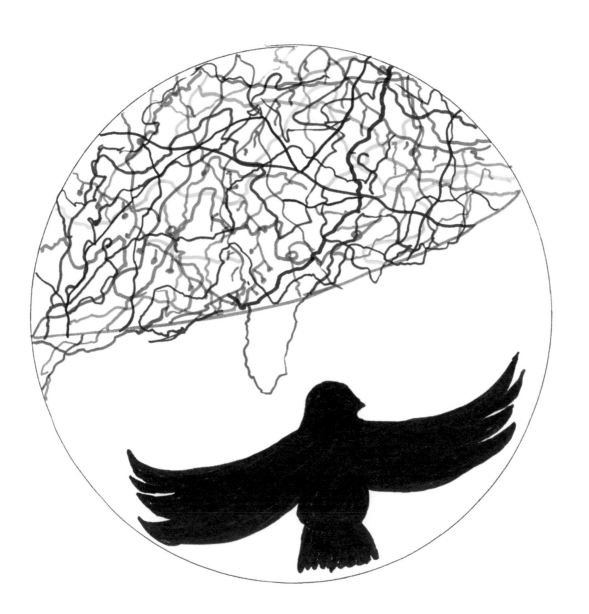

As driven as I was to do the drawings during my chemotherapy, the minute my final treatments were over, most of my drawings changed. They didn't come from the same place inside me, and I didn't have much interest in doing them. I also lost interest in my journal. It was as if there had been some benevolent guide, some spirit in the universe, who was directing the show, helping me deal with my experience of the chemotherapy. I know also that I felt as if I was a conduit—that I was making drawings whose forms were being determined by something other than my conscious mind. It was as if the drawings originated in my belly and traveled out through my arm, entirely bypassing my head and brain. I realize that my drawings and my writing came from such personal and spiritual parts of me that they did indeed serve as antidotes to the cancer and to the poison of the chemo moving through my veins—in effect, balancing the creative and destructive forces within me. My drawings felt like a mobilization of all my creative energies coming to my rescue. I can still call on them if I stay conscious and invite them to come. I forget, in the busyness of life, to remember these resources, and it is imperative that I remember. They came on their own as a gift to show me what I have.

75

POST-CHEMO, PRE-RADIATION

In early January, one week after the end of six months of chemotherapy and three weeks before the start of radiation, I managed to co-lead Woman's Way, an eight-day personal growth lab for women. Depleted as I was, I wasn't sure that I'd have enough energy to do it, but participating in this event once a year has been one of the most important parts of my personal and professional life, and I didn't want to miss it. I was especially glad that I could do it, because, for many reasons, it turned out to be the last one we would do. I spent eight days with thirty-five women, many of whom had been touched in one way or another by cancer. As I listened to their stories, some about cancer, some about illness and death, others about their own personal suffering, I felt a part of something much bigger than myself. I was part of a group of strong, wonderful women who were surviving their own hardships with great integrity and dignity. It was an extraordinarily sustaining experience for me.

FEBRUARY **13**

I went to sleep last night by the light of a very wintry moon, that moon that is carved out of such a blue, blue sky; the moon which only shines like that on a cold winter night. I woke this morning, agitated and frightened, feeling lost, strange, and very alone, even though my beloved Wheel was lying right beside me, holding my hand in his sleep. I realized that I'd been dreaming—or sleep-thinking or wake-dreaming—about death, about my body, about the mysteries of what's going on inside there, of the life of its own that this cancer has, and I found myself in a frightened victim place, a feeling that I haven't had very often since all this began.

I realized that I'd also been thinking about my dear, constant, loving but aging parents, whose lives have lost so much of their luster and for whom I wish nothing so much as peace and with whom I feel totally engaged. I felt yesterday as I looked into my old Dad's eyes and held his hand, that he was looking right into me and I into him. As I rubbed Mum's shoulders and looked into her forgetting eyes, I felt so grateful to her for her constancy and devotion. I sometimes can see their confusion as a passage, a way of disengaging, and today I'm feeling as if that disengagement is like a tunnel into whatever their next engagement may be. Other days, all I can do is rail against the indignities they're having to undergo. Then I come back to myself and where I am about my own dying, my own death, my own process.

LATER

As I've moved out of chemotherapy and into radiation, my relation to my cancer has changed, or at least my feelings about it have. I think that while chemo was ongoing, I almost felt safe, as if no cancer would dare spread with all those chemicals attacking it. I felt safe enough to imagine, to try to understand, mostly through my writing and my drawing, what was happening to me and to engage myself in healing from the inside out. I think I was in a healthy state of denial as well, not really taking in the possibility of death—at least not taking it past my head into my heart.

As I begin the radiation phase, I begin a new phase of understanding as well—understanding, mind you, without knowing anything. I'm beginning to actually hear others' stories about metastases, about more and different treatments, about death. I'm allowing myself to accept the gravity of the extent of my lymph node involvement. I'm knowing that death from this cancer is a possibility, though I'm not accepting it as an inevitability.

So, I'm in a different stage and I move from moment to moment, from a feeling of acceptance and comprehension to deep sadness to depression to a feeling of panic. Sometimes I'm grateful that I know my own body as well as I do, and sometimes, when I feel something shift or change and move immediately into "knowing" that the cancer has spread, I wish I wasn't so familiar with it.

When I woke this morning, I realized that I was hesitant to tell Wheel that I was thinking about dying. In fact, hesitant to tell anyone about it for fear of burdening them. When I did tell him, he told me I could tell him anything and I realized that by not sharing how I'm feeling I may, in fact, be keeping others from sharing their feelings with me. What makes me think I'm the only one who connects this cancer with the possibility of death?

After my radiation appointment this morning I took my first walk in a long time. I walked in the woods behind our house, a walk I've taken many times and in all seasons. It was a different walk this morning. It was so silent that I could hear everything. I could even hear the difference in the crunch of the snow between my heel and my toe hitting the ground. The first sounds I heard were bird sounds. I couldn't identify them, but it was so still that I could hear each individual song, and I had the presumptuous notion that they were singing for me, heralding spring and growth and hope. As I walked along, my step began to have some bounce in it, and I became acutely aware of every-thing I saw. The light was intense on the snow but very warm-ing. I could feel—really feel—under my feet the different tex-tures of ice, melting snow, pine needles, and dirt. Suddenly I realized that I was no longer hearing or seeing the birds and I heard myself say out loud, "Where are the birds?" Much to my astonishment, within a few seconds there were five or six chickadees flitting about the path and flying ahead of me. I felt as if I were Snow White and truly expected to see Bambi and Flower appear!

As I walked back I noticed each tree and the light playing on each one. Everything had slowed down. I felt as if I were in a time warp. By the time I got back home, I had the intense realization that those trees and those birds were as much and as important a part of the universe as I was and that I am only a tiny piece of the whole plan. I've always believed that, but this time I knew it in my body. It was such a liberating feeling that I began to feel very peaceful and happy. When I came into the house, having picked my first forsythia for forcing, I felt as if I were walking taller and more peacefully than I had in days.

It would be wrong to suggest that this last year and a half hasn't been long and often utterly debilitating, or that I haven't spent time thinking or worrying about death. In fact, I've wondered often if I'll ever be able to do things I've always wanted to do. Will this be my last Christmas? Will I see my grandchildren grow up? I have felt an urgency, a desire to not put things off until "someday." During treatments my life was so simple and I was so focused on dealing with myself and my body from moment to moment, that I didn't let myself understand the full impact of what was happening to me. I don't know what the future holds for me in terms of this cancer, but who of us does know? I will have periodic bone and CAT scans, chest X-rays, ultrasounds, and mammograms, which could pick up anything big enough to see, but otherwise, I will probably know nothing. I am taking tamoxifen, an estrogen blocker that I hope will keep the cancer from returning, but not a day goes by without my wondering what else is going on in my body. Not an ache nor a strange sensation goes on without my wondering, "Is it back again?" Since the chemo and radiation ended, I sometimes feel depressed, ungrounded, uncentered, fragmented, unsteady, unsure. It feels as if all the rules have changed, the ground has shifted, and I'm in a kind of culture shock. My world has turned upside down and isn't right side up yet.

All of these feelings and fears are balanced by my deep and abiding knowledge that I am truly blessed and sustained by my family and a community of friends who love me. I am alive and I am well today, and for that I rejoice. I know from my own experience that there is great healing power in love, in prayer, in community, in attention to quiet, in laughter, in touch, in true compassion, in the life of the spirit, in the creative process, in focusing on priorities, and in the simple life.

So, I have some choices. I can choose to live my life in anticipation of the other shoe dropping, or I can live the best way I know how: watching my diet, getting exercise and rest, laughing as much as possible and surrounding myself with people I love and who love me. The trick will be to remember what I've learned and try to live my life as fully as I can.

Walking around New York City in the rain a few weeks ago, I wandered into an interesting-looking store filled with kaleidoscopes. In the back of the store I came across a book by Shaun McNiff called *Art as Medicine*. On the back was a quote that spoke directly to what I've considered the phenomenon of my images. It explained why they came to me and why, when treatment was over, they were no longer available to me in the same way:

> *Whenever illness is associated with loss of soul, the arts emerge spontaneously as remedies, soul medicine.*

We all have our own definitions of soul, and though I had never used those words to describe my experience, in that moment I knew two things: I had associated my cancer with loss of soul and the images and drawings had emerged spontaneously as soul medicine.

Acceptance of the cancer and the months of treatment for it was as much a spiritual experience as a physical one. I didn't have the words for it then, but I felt as if the images were instructions from my core, my soul, and that putting them on paper was an imperative to my getting well.

As I write this, it is almost exactly four years since my first surgery. Happily, according to all the tests, I am healthy. I take tamoxifen twice daily and see at least one of my doctors every six months. A lot has changed in my life in those four years, including the loss of both of my parents and the arrival of three grandchildren. Several friends have died from cancer and several more are living their lives to the fullest. Life and its cycles go on around me and inside me.

Whereas I thought I would never forget the lessons I learned, it's often hard to remember to slow down and focus. I still pay relatively careful attention to my diet, exercise, and rest, but I am also increasingly aware that I am living less consciously and attentively than I was. It has taken much of this time for me to put my experience with cancer behind me and begin to look forward to the rest of my life.

83

My journal and my drawings are vivid reminders of my experience of cancer, chemotherapy, and radiation, my path through the fire. They remind me of my own inner resources, and though I do not have the dreams and images which guided me through my treatments, I know that if I needed them again they would appear as soul medicine. Looking back at my drawing of the broken porcelain cup, I realize that time has helped me fit more of the little black pieces into the jigsaw puzzle of my life, and I feel blessed beyond measure.

84

WENDY ALLEN WHEELER is a mother of four and grand-mother of five, and lives with her husband in Connecticut. While pursuing a career as a licensed clinical social worker and thera-pist/teacher, she discovered that she enjoys watercolor painting and working with clay. The spontaneous creation of the drawings in this book, however, was a mysterious process that Wendy felt compelled to begin, and continue throughout her treatment for breast cancer.

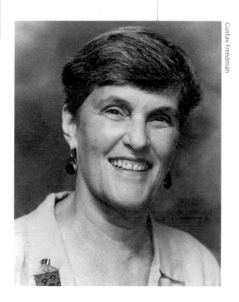

Gustav Freedman

THIS BOOK WAS SET IN JOANNA AND THESANS.